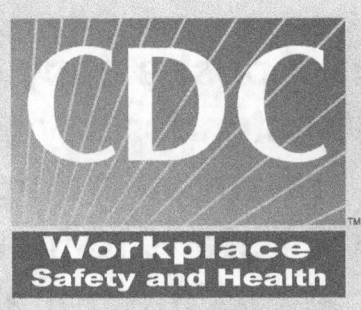

Workplace Safety and Health

Chemotherapy Drug Exposures at an Oncology Clinic – Florida

James Couch, CIH, MS, REHS/RS
Christine West, RN, MSN/MPH

Health Hazard Evaluation Report
HETA 2009-0148-3158
June 2012

DEPARTMENT OF HEALTH AND HUMAN SERVICES
Centers for Disease Control and Prevention

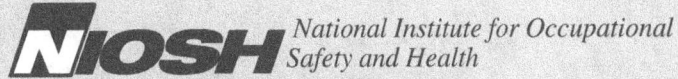

National Institute for Occupational Safety and Health

The employer shall post a copy of this report for a period of 30 calendar days at or near the workplace(s) of affected employees. The employer shall take steps to insure that the posted determinations are not altered, defaced, or covered by other material during such period. [37 FR 23640, November 7, 1972, as amended at 45 FR 2653, January 14, 1980].

CONTENTS

ABBREVIATIONS

ACGIH®	American Conference of Governmental Industrial Hygienists
ASHP	American Society of Health-System Pharmacists
BSC	Biological safety cabinet
BVNA	Bureau Veritas North America
CDC	Centers for Disease Control and Prevention
CFR	Code of Federal Regulations
cm	Centimeter
cm^2	Centimeter squared
HEPA	High-efficiency particulate air
HHE	Health hazard evaluation
IARC	International Agency for Research on Cancer
IV	Intravenous
LOD	Limit of detection
LOQ	Limit of quantitation
NAICS	North American Industry Classification System
NIOSH	National Institute for Occupational Safety and Health
ng	Nanogram
$ng/100\ cm^2$	Nanograms per 100 square centimeters
OEL	Occupational exposure limit
OSHA	Occupational Safety and Health Administration
PEL	Permissible exposure limit
PPE	Personal protective equipment
REL	Recommended exposure limit
STEL	Short-term exposure limit
TLV®	Threshold limit value
TWA	Time-weighted average
WEEL™	Workplace environmental exposure level
USP	United States Pharmacopeia

The National Institute for Occupational Safety and Health (NIOSH) received a confidential employee request for a health hazard evaluation (HHE) at an oncology clinic in Florida. Employees submitting the HHE request were concerned with work-related upper respiratory irritation, headache, fainting, diarrhea, loss of appetite, and other health effects.

What NIOSH Did

- We evaluated the clinic in September 2009 and November 2010.

- We took surface wipe samples for platinum-containing chemotherapy drugs during the first and second visits. During the second visit we also tested for cyclophosphamide, ifosfamide, and doxorubicin.

- We took hand wipe samples for platinum-containing chemotherapy drugs during the first site visit. The samples were from two nurses who had recently handled these drugs.

- We checked the air flow of the biological safety cabinet.

- We talked with employees about their health and safety concerns.

- We reviewed work-related injuries and illnesses for 2006 through 2008.

What NIOSH Found

- Platinum-containing chemotherapy drugs were found in most of the surface wipe samples.

- No platinum-containing chemotherapy drugs were found in the hand wipe samples.

- Cyclophosphamide and ifosfamide were found in some surface wipe samples.

- The biological safety cabinet operated properly and was checked annually.

- The most commonly reported health concerns were upper respiratory symptoms.

- Employees reported inconsistent use of personal protective equipment. They also reported that training on the occupational hazards of chemotherapy drugs was not sufficient.

What Managers Can Do

- Review the cleaning procedures with the staff on how chemotherapy drugs should be handled.

- Observe employee and patient activities in the checkout area to find where chemotherapy drug cross-contamination may occur.

- Instruct employees and cleaning staff to clean work surfaces after chemotherapy drugs are used and at the end of each day.

HIGHLIGHTS OF THE NIOSH HEALTH HAZARD EVALUATION (CONTINUED)

- Start a health and safety committee that includes managers and employees to routinely discuss health and safety concerns.

- Start a medical surveillance program, and provide annual training for staff who handle chemotherapy drugs.

- Require that employees wear gowns, goggles, and double chemotherapy protective gloves when preparing and administering chemotherapy drugs.

What Employees Can Do

- Wear all required personal protective equipment when preparing and handling chemotherapy drugs.

- Carry chemotherapy drugs in a sealed outer container to prevent spills.

- Clean up any chemotherapy drugs spills quickly using the proper spill kit.

- Dispose of chemotherapy drugs and any disposable administration equipment in yellow chemotherapy waste bags.

- Report all symptoms that you think are related to work. Follow-up with a healthcare provider who is knowledgeable about occupational diseases.

- Report any workplace safety or health concerns to your supervisor.

NIOSH investigators evaluated potential occupational exposures to chemotherapy drugs at an oncology clinic. We sampled for platinum-containing chemotherapy drugs, cyclophosphamide, ifosfamide, and doxorubicin on surfaces. We found platinum-containing chemotherapy drugs and cyclophosphamide and ifosfamide. We recommend that the clinic review cleaning practices and PPE use to reduce employee exposures to chemotherapy drugs.

On May 1, 2009, NIOSH received a confidential employee request for an HHE at an oncology clinic in Florida. The request concerned potential exposures to chemotherapy drugs and adverse health effects such as upper respiratory symptoms, rash, diarrhea, migraine, and headache. During our first site visit in September 2009, we measured the face velocity of the Class 2 BSC where chemotherapy drugs were mixed and collected surface and hand wipe samples for platinum-containing chemotherapy drugs. We also conducted health interviews with 14 of 54 employees and reviewed the OSHA Form 300 Log of Work-Related Injuries and Illnesses for 2006 through 2008.

In November 2010, during our second evaluation, we collected surface wipe samples (but no hand wipe samples) for platinum-containing chemotherapy drugs in similar locations as in the 2009 evaluation. We also collected surface wipe samples for cyclophosphamide, ifosfamide, and doxorubicin at the beginning of the work day before the chemotherapy drugs were unpacked and at the end of the work day after the last chemotherapy treatment was completed. We did this to evaluate the clinic's cleaning procedures and employee work practices.

Platinum-containing chemotherapy drugs were detected in most surface wipe samples during both evaluations but not on the two hand wipes collected in 2009 from nurses who had recently handled platinum-containing chemotherapy drugs. Cyclophosphamide and ifosfamide were detected on surface wipe samples collected throughout the clinic, suggesting inadequate work practices and housekeeping. Doxorubicin was not detected on any surface wipe samples but its recovery may have been poor because these wipe samples had been frozen for approximately 7 months awaiting development of an analytical method [Burr 2011a].

The Class 2 BSC was certified biannually. The sash alarm that was malfunctioning during our first visit had been repaired by our second visit. The average BSC face velocity we measured was 275 feet per minute, which met the CDC recommendation of at least 100 feet per minute [CDC 2007].

Of the 14 employees we interviewed, 4 reported health symptoms consisting of runny nose, sneezing, eye irritation, and headache that improved on their days off work. One of these four reported a recurring "burning" rash on his nose after handling chemotherapy drug waste. All interviewed employees reported

SUMMARY
(CONTINUED)

adequate training about the safe preparation, administration, and disposal of chemotherapy drugs. However, three employees reported inadequate training on the potential short- and long-term health effects of chemotherapy drug exposure. When preparing chemotherapy drugs, all employees reported using double gloves, goggles, and chemotherapy protective gowns. Some employees stated they voluntarily wore disposable filtering facepiece respirators and/or surgical masks to avoid contaminating the chemotherapy drugs and/or to protect the patients. Four employees reported not consistently double gloving or using chemotherapy protective gowns when administering chemotherapy drugs to patients. Some employees also reported reusing disposable surgical masks.

Considering the inconsistent use of PPE and presence of chemotherapy drug residue in the clinic work area, employees are at risk of both acute and chronic health effects from exposure to chemotherapy drugs. We recommend the clinic improve employee work practices and housekeeping, start a medical surveillance program for employees, provide annual training, and require the use of appropriate PPE when handling chemotherapy drugs.

Keywords: NAICS 621111 Office of Physicians (Except Mental Health Specialists), anti-neoplastic drugs, cisplatin, cyclophosphamide, ifosfamide, doxorubicin, healthcare personnel, chemotherapy drugs, housekeeping

INTRODUCTION

In May 2009, NIOSH received a confidential employee request for an HHE at an oncology clinic ("clinic") in Florida. The HHE request was submitted because of concerns about potential exposures to chemotherapy drugs and suspected associated adverse health effects such as upper respiratory symptoms, rash, diarrhea, migraine, and headache.

NIOSH investigators conducted a site visit on September 21–22, 2009. We held an opening meeting with clinic managers and employee representatives to discuss the HHE request, health concerns, and the scope of the evaluation. We collected surface and hand wipe samples for platinum-containing chemotherapy drugs (such as cisplatin, a chemotherapy drug frequently administered at the clinic). Employees also participated in confidential health interviews. A closing meeting was held on September 22, 2009, with employer and employee representatives to summarize our site visit activities and provide preliminary findings. On the basis of initial sample results we visited the clinic again on November 15–18, 2010, to collect additional surface wipe samples (but no hand wipe samples) for platinum-containing chemotherapy drugs and for cyclophosphamide, ifosfamide, and doxorubicin (other chemotherapy drugs used at the clinic).

In an interim letter to employer and employee representatives dated April 8, 2010, we provided our preliminary recommendations and reported the hand and surface wipe sample results collected in September 2009. Because we had described these results as measurements of cisplatin in a February 11, 2011 letter, we recalculated and reported the wipe sample results as platinum. Several platinum-containing chemotherapy drugs (not just cisplatin) were used at the clinic. Our surface wipe samples were analyzed only for total platinum, not for any specific platinum-containing chemotherapy drug. In this final report all hand and surface wipe samples that were collected for platinum-containing chemotherapy drugs are reported as platinum. Results of the surface wipe sample results we collected in November 2010 for cyclophosphamide, ifosfamide, and doxorubicin were not available at the time of the February 2011 letter because these analyses were delayed by the need to develop an analytical method.

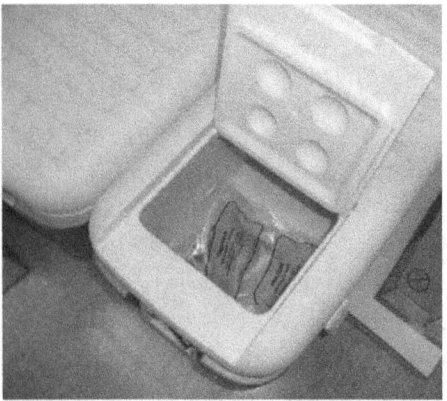

Figure 1. Each morning a local pharmacy delivered chemotherapy drugs in coolers, which were stored in the pharmacy room.

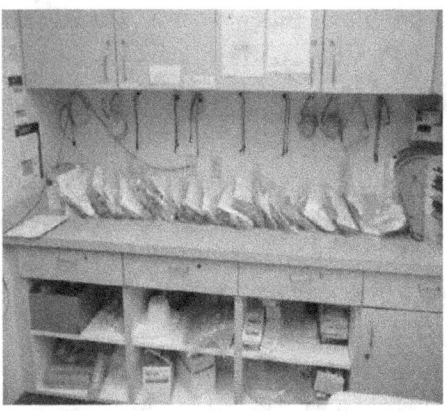

Figure 2. Chemotherapy drug bags were stored on a counter in the clinic pharmacy along with personal protective equipment.

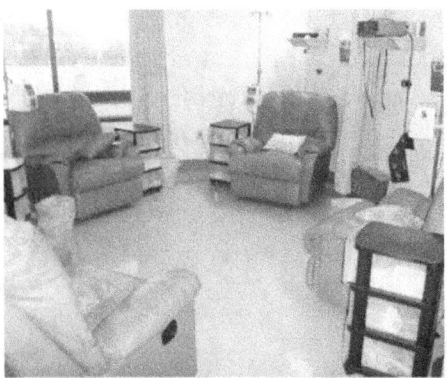

Figure 3. One of two chemotherapy administration rooms used by patients.

Work Process

Chemotherapy drugs were delivered to the clinic in coolers from a local pharmacy and received by the clinic's pharmacy (Figure 1). These chemotherapy drugs were double-bagged, and the descriptions of the contents were clearly visible without opening the bag. Some of these drugs were mixed in the clinic pharmacy because of the drug's short half-life.

A clinic pharmacy employee emptied the coolers and arranged the bagged drugs chronologically on a countertop according to the patient's appointment (Figure 2). All employees handling chemotherapy drugs were required to wear two pairs of chemotherapy protective gloves (double-gloving), and some tasks also required wearing a chemotherapy protective apron. Some employees stated they voluntarily wore disposable surgical masks to avoid contaminating the chemotherapy drugs and/or to protect the patients. Upon patient arrival, nurses retrieved the appropriate chemotherapy bag from the pharmacy and transported it to one of two treatment rooms.

After verifying the chemotherapy drug treatment with the patient's medical record, a nurse began administration via an IV bag hung from a stand adjacent to the patient chair. The chemotherapy drug administration time varied from minutes to hours depending on the treatment protocol (Figure 3).

After completing the chemotherapy treatment the nurse removed the IV from the patient and disposed of all the chemotherapy drug-contaminated materials in a chemotherapy waste container. The nurse then removed both pairs of chemotherapy protective gloves and placed them in the chemotherapy waste container. The patient was then escorted to the checkout area for discharge.

Surface and Hand Wipe Samples

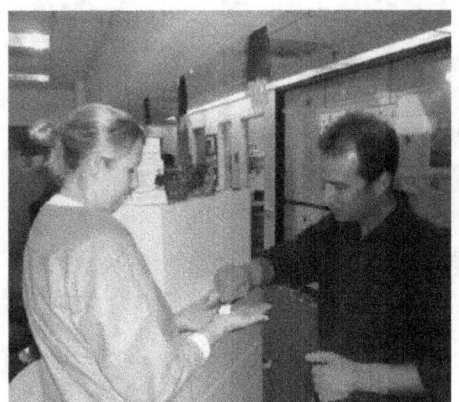

Figure 4. NIOSH investigator collecting a hand wipe sample from a nurse after she administered a chemotherapy drug.

In the September 2009 evaluation, we collected surface and hand wipe samples for platinum-containing chemotherapy drugs and analyzed the samples for total platinum (Figure 4). We used professional judgment to select sample locations where clinic employees handled or administered chemotherapy drugs. In the November 2010 evaluation, we collected surface wipe (but no hand wipe) samples for platinum-containing chemotherapy drugs in similar locations as in the 2009 evaluation. However, in the November 2010 evaluation we sampled for cyclophosphamide, ifosfamide, and doxorubicin at the beginning of the work day before these chemotherapy drugs were unpacked and again after the last chemotherapy treatment was completed but before the housekeeping staff arrived for the overnight cleaning. The intent of collecting these morning and evening surface wipe samples was to help evaluate the effectiveness of the overnight housekeeping procedures in removing residual chemotherapy drugs from surfaces in the clinic. Figure 5 illustrates collecting a surface wipe sample on the work surface of the Class 2 BSC using a sample template. Appendix A describes the surface and hand wipe sampling methods used in this evaluation for platinum-containing chemotherapy drugs, cyclophosphamide, ifosfamide, and doxorubicin.

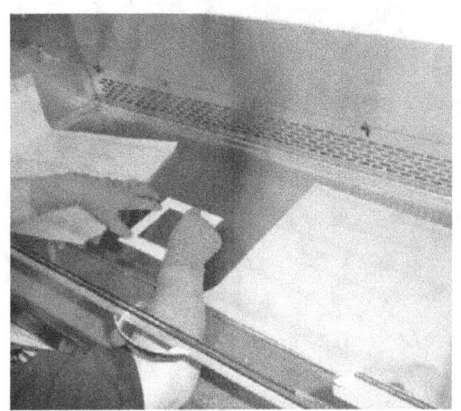

Figure 5. NIOSH investigator using a sampling template to collect a surface wipe sample inside the Class 2 BSC.

To assess environmental exposures to platinum-containing chemotherapy agents such as cisplatin, carboplatin, and oxaliplatin, we sampled for platinum, a metal not typically present in the environment. Because several platinum-containing chemotherapy agents were used at the clinic, this sampling approach did not allow us to specifically identify the chemotherapy agent that may have been the source of the platinum. However, it did allow us to indirectly measure platinum-containing chemotherapy agents on surfaces in the clinic and thus to evaluate the efficacy of engineering and administrative controls, work practices, and housekeeping in minimizing employee exposures. Appendix B discusses the OELs and health effects of chemotherapy drugs.

Health Interviews and Review of Injury/illness Records

We selected a convenience sample of 10 clinical and 4 administration staff among the 54 employees who were present on September 21–22, 2009, for health interviews. We asked about procedures for handling and administering chemotherapy drugs, acute and chronic health symptoms potentially associated with chemotherapy drugs, personal cancer history, reproductive health, use of PPE, and workplace health and safety training. We reviewed OSHA Form 300 Log of Work-Related Injuries and Illnesses for years 2006 through 2008.

Biological Safety Cabinet Evaluation

We observed employees using the Class 2 BSC, reviewed the biannual certification records, and asked staff and managers about the performance and operating procedures for the BSC. The BSC had a HEPA filter and exhausted 100% of the captured air outside the clinic. We used a thermal anemometer to evaluate the face velocity of the BSC (Appendix A).

Review of Housekeeping Practices

A third-party contractor performed housekeeping duties after the clinic closed. Although we did not observe the housekeeping staff performing their duties, we reviewed their procedures and discussed the housekeeping practices with the clinic management and employees.

Surface and Hand Wipe Samples

We detected platinum in 18 of the 26 surface wipe samples (69%) collected during our September 2009 evaluation (Appendix C, Table C1). Of the 18 wipe samples that contained platinum, 14 had levels that ranged between the LOD and LOQ, meaning some uncertainty was associated with the quantitative results. The highest level we measured, 91 ng/100 cm^2, was collected in the clinic pharmacy on the floor in front of the BSC. We did not detect platinum (<0.7 ng /sample) in either of two hand wipe samples collected from two nurses who had recently administered chemotherapy drugs.

We detected platinum in 16 of the 20 surface wipe samples (80%) collected during our November 2010 evaluation. Two of the 16 wipe samples (12%) had levels that were between the LOD and the LOQ. The highest surface wipe levels were collected in the clinic pharmacy (12 ng/100 cm^2, on the middle of the BSC work surface) and in the right treatment room (13 ng/100 cm^2, on the countertop next to the sink in the bedroom).

Surface wipe samples detected cyclophosphamide and ifosfamide in the clinic pharmacy, left and right treatment rooms, and the checkout area. The highest level of cyclophosphamide (28,000 ng/100 cm^2) was measured in the left treatment room underneath the IV stand. Every sample collected for cyclophosphamide from underneath the IV stand in the left treatment room was detected above the LOQ of 17 ng/sample. All detectable ifosfamide levels (two samples from the floor in front of the BSC in the clinic pharmacy) were between the LOD and the LOQ. No other sample locations had detectable ifosfamide levels. Doxorubicin was not detected (LOD = 7 ng/sample) in any of the surface wipe samples collected in the clinic. However, the recovery of doxorubicin may have been poor because the wipe samples were frozen for 7 months prior to analysis (see Discussion). Appendix C, Table C2 contains detailed sample results for cyclophosphamide; Appendix C, Table C3 contains the detailed sample results for ifosfamide.

Health Interviews and Review of Injury/ illness Records

The average employment of the 14 employees we interviewed (10 clinical and 4 administrative staff) at the clinic was 7 years. Nine clinical staff reported handling chemotherapy drugs; of these employees, five reported preparing and administering IV drugs. Four employees reported health symptoms consisting of runny nose, sneezing, eye irritation, and headache that improved on their days off work. One of the four employees reported a recurring "burning" rash on his nose after handling chemotherapy drug waste. None of the employees interviewed reported a history of cancer or reproductive health problems. Employees reported adequate training about the safe preparation, administration, and disposal of chemotherapy drugs; however, a few employees reported inadequate training on the potential risk of short- and long-term health effects of chemotherapy drug exposure.

Of the entries for injuries or illnesses on the OSHA Logs from 2006 through 2008, one entry was recorded for burn from intravenous tubing, one for skin rash, and five for needlestick injuries. As determined in discussions with managers and employees, no medical surveillance program existed at the clinic that was specific to chemotherapy drug exposure.

Other Workplace Observations

When preparing chemotherapy drugs, all clinic employees reported using gloves, goggles, and chemotherapy protective gowns. However, we observed some employees not consistently double gloving or using chemotherapy protective gowns when handling or administering chemotherapy drugs. Specifically, one employee was observed handling a chemotherapy drug and using her gloved hand to brush her hair away from her eyes. Another employee was carrying chemotherapy drugs in her arms and against her body, but was not wearing a chemotherapy protective gown or carrying a spill kit. These work practices increase the risk of getting chemotherapy drugs on clothing or skin.

Four employees reported voluntarily wearing and reusing disposable filtering facepiece respirators and/or surgical masks and changing them once per week. According to the employees, the respirators and surgical masks were worn to lessen the chance of contaminating the chemotherapy drugs and the patients. We observed what appeared to be dirt around the nose area of some of these respirators and surgical masks. Additionally, some of these employees improperly stored their respirators and surgical masks by hanging them on hooks directly over the chemotherapy drug bags and plastic containers used to transport the chemotherapy drugs to the patient (Figure 2).

We observed containers of bleach and alcohol stored in the clinic pharmacy that did not have hazard warning information as required by the OSHA hazard communication standard [29 CFR 1910.1200]. We also observed food stored on a counter that was also used to prepare chemotherapy drug doses.

Biological Safety Cabinet Face Velocity

The average face velocity (275 feet per minute) of the Class 2 BSC met the CDC recommendation of at least 100 feet per minute [CDC 2007]. The sash alarm that worked intermittently during our initial visit had been repaired. However, the BSC was not physically marked to indicate a hood sash location that would ensure at least 100 feet per minute of air flow.

Housekeeping Practices

During our interviews, employees and the employer expressed concerns that housekeeping practices related to cleaning and disposal of chemotherapy drug waste were inadequate. One employee reported that during the day shift, chemotherapy drug waste containers were not regularly emptied; this employee was concerned about exposure to contaminated equipment.

DISCUSSION

We found platinum in several of our surface wipe samples, demonstrating that employees may be exposed to platinum-containing chemotherapy drugs, including cisplatin. Other researchers have found platinum contamination in pharmacies [Brouwers et al. 2007]. Currently no OELs exist for platinum-containing chemotherapy drugs on surfaces or in the air. However, considering the carcinogenicity of these chemotherapy drugs [IARC 2004] it would be prudent to maintain exposures as low as reasonably achievable.

During the November 2010 site visit we detected cyclophosphamide in the clinic pharmacy (on the floor in front of the BSC and the prepared drugs), the left treatment room (under the IV stand next to the first chair), and the checkout (desk surface on the right). The highest level (28,000 ng/100 cm²) was found in the left treatment room beneath an IV stand. Although no spills or accidents were reported, it is possible that there may have been surface contamination or an undetected leak on the IV bag. The results from surface samples collected at this location over the following 2 days of the November 2010 evaluation were also among the highest we collected, suggesting that cyclophosphamide is stable in the environment and that housekeeping procedures were not effectively removing this chemotherapy drug in one cleaning. The NIOSH Alert on handling chemotherapy drugs provides detailed information on housekeeping and cleaning procedures to effectively and promptly remove these drugs from work surfaces [NIOSH 2004].

Cyclophosphamide was detected in every surface wipe sample collected in the checkout area. Although most of these results were between the LOD and the LOQ, the presence of cyclophosphamide is significant because no chemotherapy drugs were administered in the checkout area. As such, the clinic employees in this area did not wear PPE, and patients in the checkout area could unknowingly have been exposed to chemotherapy drugs that were not in their oncology drug treatment protocols. Additionally, family members and the general public in the checkout area could have been exposed to chemotherapy drugs. We did not identify the source of the chemotherapy drugs in the checkout area but contaminated paperwork, contaminated skin of employees, or the patients themselves, may have been possible sources.

Although we detected cyclophosphamide and ifosfamide, we did not detect doxorubicin. The surface wipe samples for these drugs were kept frozen for approximately 7 months while an analytical method was developed. NIOSH has conducted stability studies of cyclophosphamide and ifosfamide when collected on surface wipe samples, and no degradation of recovery was observed [Burr 2011a]. However, NIOSH chemists have observed in laboratory experiments that doxorubicin degraded after being frozen [Burr 2011b]. Therefore, we cannot exclude the possibility that doxorubicin may have been present when the surface wipe samples were collected.

Upper respiratory symptoms and rash that were worse at work were reported by four clinic employees. Given the inconsistent use of PPE reported and evidence of chemotherapy drug residue in the work environment, employees were at risk of acute and chronic health effects from exposure to chemotherapy drugs. Occupational exposures to chemotherapy drugs can lead to acute effects such as skin rash and upper respiratory irritation [McDiarmid and Egan 1988; Krstev et al. 2003; NIOSH 2004]. However, other factors that we did not account for, such as use of latex gloves and hospital cleaning solutions in the workplace, may cause upper respiratory symptoms and rash. Therefore, because of the small number of employees reporting symptoms and the nonspecific nature of these symptoms, we cannot determine if they are directly related to chemotherapy drug exposures from this evaluation. Chronic health effects known to be associated with exposure to chemotherapy drugs are cancer and adverse reproductive health outcomes, and they may not manifest until later in life [Skov et al. 1992; Valanis et al. 1999; Harrison 2001; Krstev et al. 2003; NIOSH 2004].

The typical routes of exposure to chemotherapy drugs in healthcare settings are inhalation, dermal, and oral. Inhalation exposure may occur from airborne droplets, vapors, or dust generated by crushing tablets. Dermal exposure may occur when employees touch contaminated surfaces during the preparation, administration, or disposal of chemotherapy drugs, and oral exposure may occur from hand-to mouth contact. Accidental injection with a chemotherapy drug, although rare, has been documented [Connor and McDiarmid 2008] and this may be a source of exposure for the employees given past incidents of needlestick injuries recorded on the OSHA Logs. We did not evaluate or observe any activities during our evaluation that should require the use of respiratory protection.

Conclusions

We found chemotherapy drugs in surface wipe samples collected throughout the clinic, and cyclophosphamide was found in checkout, an area that should not have any chemotherapy drug contamination. One sample location remained positive for cyclophosphamide throughout our 3 day November 2010 evaluation, suggesting that housekeeping procedures were not effectively removing this chemotherapy drug in one cleaning. Upper respiratory symptoms were the most commonly reported among clinic employees but because these are nonspecific and common in the general population we do not know whether these symptoms are associated with chemotherapy drug exposures. Our findings suggest that employees are at risk from exposure to chemotherapy drugs, that employee work procedures can be improved, and that housekeeping practices were insufficient in removing some chemotherapy drugs from contaminated surfaces.

Recommendations

On the basis of our findings, we recommend the actions listed below to create a more healthful workplace. We encourage the clinic to use a labor-management health and safety committee or working group to discuss the recommendations in this report and develop an action plan. Those involved in the work can best set priorities and assess the feasibility of our recommendations for the specific situation at the clinic. Our recommendations are based on the hierarchy of controls approach (Appendix B: Occupational Exposure Limits and Health Effects). This approach groups actions by their likely effectiveness in reducing or removing hazards. In most cases, the preferred approach is to eliminate hazardous materials or processes and install engineering controls to reduce exposure or shield employees. Until such controls are in place, or if they are not effective or feasible, administrative measures and/or PPE may be needed.

Engineering Controls

Engineering controls reduce exposures to employees by removing the hazard from the process or placing a barrier between the hazard and the employee. Engineering controls are very effective at protecting employees without placing primary responsibility of implementation on the employee.

1. Transport chemotherapy drug bags and related equipment to the administration area in plastic bins to minimize contact with potentially contaminated surfaces. The plastic bin should be cleaned after each use.

2. Mark the BSC sash height that would ensure at least 100 feet per minute of air flow.

Administrative Controls

Administrative controls are management-dictated work practices and policies to reduce or prevent exposures to workplace hazards. The effectiveness of administrative changes in work practices for controlling workplace hazards is dependent on both employer commitment and employee acceptance. Regular monitoring and reinforcement are necessary to ensure that control policies and procedures are not circumvented in the name of convenience or production.

1. Review policies and procedures, with participation from employee and employer representatives, of the clinic's program for the safe handling and control of chemotherapy and other hazardous drugs. On the basis of this review, implement a hazard communication (worker and employer right-to know) program for any hazardous chemicals that are used in the clinic. The OSHA hazard communication standard (CFR 29, Part 1910.1200 [36]) provides information essential to establishing and maintaining a safe and healthful work environment, including:

   a. creating a worksite health hazards inventory
   b. informing employees about the hazardous compounds present and how to handle them
   c. labeling all containers with the identity of the contents and with appropriate hazard warning information

2. Provide additional training to clinic employees on the proper procedures for handling chemotherapy drugs, wearing PPE, using BSCs, cleaning, housekeeping, disposing of chemotherapy drugs, and responding to spills. The training should also include a hands-on component to demonstrate proficiency. For example, test kits using fluorescein dye could help assess techniques of clinic employees who prepare, handle, or clean-up chemotherapy drugs. This training should be conducted upon hire before beginning duties and at least yearly (or more often if deficiencies are observed). Competency testing should be performed to evaluate training effectiveness [USP 2008].

3. Offer duty-specific training on the potential health and reproductive effects of chemotherapy drugs for exposed employees in receiving, transport, pharmacy preparation, administration, nursing, housekeeping, and disposal. The

level of detail and complexity of the training should be tailored to the specific job area.

4. Start a medical surveillance program for staff handling chemotherapy drugs. Establish and maintain a confidential database with information regarding each employee's medical history, with linkage to exposure information. The database should include results of a general health questionnaire, complete blood count and urinalysis, physical examination at time of employment and annually, and follow-up for employees who have shown health changes [Connor and McDiarmid 2008]. Additional information on developing a medical surveillance program for employees exposed to chemotherapy drugs can be found in NIOSH guidelines at http://www.cdc.gov/niosh/docs/wp-solutions/2007-117 and OSHA guidelines at http://www.osha.gov/dts/osta/otm/otm_vi/otm_vi_2.html#6 [OSHA 1999; NIOSH 2007]. The medical surveillance program should include:

a. A general health and reproductive health questionnaire, completed upon hire, periodically (such as yearly), and at job termination or transfer. The health questionnaires and laboratory tests (recommended below) should be evaluated for trends that may indicate health changes due to chemotherapy drug exposure.

b. A complete blood count with differential and reticulocyte count should be performed as an indicator of bone marrow reserve upon hire, periodically (such as yearly), and at job termination or transfer. Additional tests such as liver function and transaminase should also be considered, particularly if employees are exposed to agents considered hepatotoxic. Urine should be monitored periodically by urine dipstick or microscopic examination for blood, as several chemotherapy drugs (such as cyclophosphamide) are known to cause bladder damage and blood in the urine of treated patients.

c. A physical exam should be completed upon hire or before assuming duties with chemotherapy drugs to establish a baseline for comparison and when indicated based on abnormal results from health questionnaire, urinalysis, or blood work.

RECOMMENDATIONS (CONTINUED)

d. A follow-up medical exam should be provided if employees have health changes or have experienced a significant exposure to chemotherapy drugs, such as from a large spill, substantial skin exposure, etc.

e. Based on OSHA Technical Manual, TED 1-0.15A, Section VI, Chapter 2. Controlling Occupational Exposure to Hazardous Drugs, no biological monitoring tests (such as genotoxic markers) are currently recommended for routine use in employee medical surveillance programs [OSHA 1999].

5. Establish and clearly communicate with the cleaning contractor the janitorial policies and procedures for each clinic area where chemotherapy drugs are handled.

6. Observe patient and paperwork activities in the checkout area to identify potential sources of chemotherapy drug contamination.

7. Clean the BSCs with a deactivating agent and disinfectant at the beginning and end of the shift, before and after each activity, and after spills. The ASHP notes that strong oxidizing agents such as sodium hypochlorite solution may effectively deactivate many chemotherapy drugs [ASHP 2006]. Because of the corrosive nature of sodium hypochlorite on surfaces, using a thiosulfate-based solution after cleaning with sodium hypochlorite can help to neutralize its effect. The USP guidelines require a final cleaning with a residue-free disinfecting agent, such as sterile 70% isopropyl alcohol [USP 2008].

8. Sample work surfaces in the clinic periodically for chemotherapy drugs. Although NIOSH and OSHA do not have OELs for surface levels of chemotherapy drugs, periodic sampling would allow comparisons over time to help evaluate the effectiveness of employee work practices, administrative controls, and housekeeping.

9. Encourage employees to report all health concerns to their supervisors. These employees should be evaluated by consulting healthcare providers knowledgeable about occupational diseases.

10. Prohibit the consumption of food or beverages in work areas where chemotherapy drugs are handled.

Personal Protective Equipment

PPE is the least effective means for controlling employee exposures. Proper use of PPE requires a comprehensive program, and calls for a high level of employee involvement and commitment to be effective. The use of PPE requires the choice of the appropriate equipment to reduce the hazard and the development of supporting programs such as training, change-out schedules, and medical assessment if needed. PPE should not be relied upon as the sole method for limiting employee exposures. Rather, PPE should be used until engineering and administrative controls can be demonstrated to be effective in limiting exposures to acceptable levels.

1. Ensure that appropriate PPE (chemotherapy protective gloves, gowns, and protective eyewear) is readily available in work areas where exposure to chemotherapy drugs may occur. Gloves used should be tested and certified by the American Society for Testing and Materials for use against chemotherapy drugs [ASTM 2005] and should be labeled as chemotherapy gloves. Because of the risk for latex sensitivity, it is preferable to use nonlatex chemotherapy protective gloves. Gloves should be changed every 30 minutes or when torn, punctured, or contaminated. Employees should wash their hands immediately after gloves are removed. Protective gowns should be disposable and made of polyethylene-coated polypropylene (nonlinting and nonabsorbent) or other laminate materials. Gowns should have closed fronts, long sleeves, and elastic or knit closed cuffs. Dispose of gowns after each use. Eye and face protection should be worn whenever there is the potential for chemotherapy drugs to splash in the face or eyes.

2. Double glove with chemotherapy protective gloves when processing, preparing, administering, cleaning, or otherwise handling chemotherapy drugs.

3. Follow the OSHA respiratory protection standard [29 CFR 1910.134] regarding voluntary use of respirators, including providing Appendix D of the OSHA respiratory protection standard [29 CFR 1910.134] to employees.

4. Require employees voluntarily wearing respirators to store them properly and to replace them when they become visibly clogged or difficult to breathe through.

REFERENCES

American Society of Health-System Pharmacists [2006]. ASHP Guidelines on Handling Hazardous Drugs. Am J Health Sys Pharm 63(12): 1172-1193.

ASTM [2005]. ASTM D6978-05 Standard Practice for Assessment of Resistance of Medical Gloves to Permeation by Chemotherapy Drugs. West Conshohocken, PA: American Society for Testing and Materials International.

Brouwers, E, Huitema A, Bakker E, Douma J, Schimmel K, Weringh G, de Wolf P, Schellens J, Beijnen J [2007]. Monitoring of platinum surface contamination in seven Dutch hospital pharmacies using inductively coupled plasma mass spectrometry. Int Arch Occup Environ Health 80(8):689-699.

Burr G [2011a]. E-mail on October 7, 2011, between G. Burr, Division of Surveillance, Hazard Evaluations and Field Studies and J. Pretty, Division of Applied Research and Technology, National Institute for Occupational Safety and Health, Centers for Disease Control and Prevention, U.S. Department of Health and Human Services.

Burr G [2011b]. Personal communication on September 29, 2011, between G. Burr, Division of Surveillance, Hazard Evaluations and Field Studies and J. Pretty, Division of Applied Research and Technology, National Institute for Occupational Safety and Health, Centers for Disease Control and Prevention, U.S. Department of Health and Human Services.

CDC [2007]. Primary containment for biohazards: selection, installation and use of biological safety cabinets, 3rd edition. [http://www.cdc.gov/od/ohs/biosfty/primary_containment_for_biohazards.pdf]. Date accessed: March 2012.

CFR. Code of Federal Regulations. Washington, DC: U.S. Government Printing Office, Office of the Federal Register.

Connor TH, McDiarmid MA [2008]. Preventing occupational exposures to antineoplastic drugs in health care settings. CA Cancer J Clin 56(6):354-365.

Harrison BR [2001]. Risks of handling cytotoxic drugs. In: Perry MC ed., The chemotherapy source book. 3rd ed. Philadelphia, PA: Lippincott, Williams and Wilkins, pp. 566–582.

IARC [2004]. IARC monographs on the evaluation of the carcinogenic risk of chemicals to humans. Lyons, France: World Health Organization, International Agency for Research on Cancer. [http://monographs.iarc.fr/]. Date accessed: March 2012.

Krstev S, Perunicic B, Vidakovic A [2003]. Work practice and some adverse health effects in nurses handling antineoplastic drugs. Med Lav 94(5):432-439.

McDiarmid M, Egan T [1988]. Acute occupational exposure to antineoplastic agents J Occup Med 35(12):984-987.

NIOSH [2004]. NIOSH alert: preventing occupational exposures to antineoplastic and other hazardous drugs in health care settings. Cincinnati, OH: U.S. Department of Health and Human Services, Centers for Disease Control and Prevention, National Institute for Occupational Safety and Health, DHHS (NIOSH) Publication No. 2004-165.

NIOSH [2007]. Workplace solutions: medical surveillance for healthcare workers exposed to hazardous drugs. Cincinnati, OH: U.S. Department of Health and Human Services, Centers for Disease Control and Prevention, National Institute for Occupational Safety and Health, DHHS (NIOSH) Publication No. 2007-117.

OSHA [1999]. Technical Manual: controlling occupational exposure to hazardous drugs, Section V1 Chapter 2. Occupational Safety and Health Administration, Washington DC: TED 01-00-015. U.S. Government Printing Office.

Skov T, Maarup B, Olsen J, Rørth M, Winthereik H, Lynge E [1992]. Leukaemia and reproductive outcome among nurses handling antineoplastic drugs. Br J Ind Med 49(12):855–861.

USP [2008]. Chapter 797, Pharmaceutical compoundings – sterile preparations. Rockville, MD: United States Pharmacopeia and National Formulary.

Valanis B, Vollmer WM, Steele P [1999]. Occupational exposure to antineoplastic agents: self-reported miscarriages and stillbirths among nurses and pharmacists. J Occup Environ Med 41(8):632–638.

Surface and Hand Wipe Samples for Platinum-containing Chemotherapy Drugs

Surface and hand wipe samples were taken using Alpha Texwipe swabs moistened with deionized water. For surfaces we used a 10 cm × 10 cm disposable template to determine the sampling area. For hand wipes we held the moistened sample media with forceps while wiping the employee's hands. For each wipe sample we wore a clean pair of chemotherapy–drug-resistant gloves. The wipe sample media were analyzed for platinum by inductively coupled plasma/mass spectrometry. For the samples collected during the September 2009 evaluation, the LOD was 0.7 ng platinum per sample, and the LOQ was 9.8 ng of platinum per sample. The LOD was 0.3 ng platinum per sample, and the LOQ was 0.84 ng platinum per sample for the samples collected during the November 2010 evaluation. For both evaluations the sampling and analytical method for measuring platinum in surface and hand wipe samples was developed by Bureau Veritas North America.

Surface Samples for Cyclophosphamide, Ifosfamide, and Doxorubicin

Each surface wipe sample was collected using two Whatman filters (42 millimeter diameter) moistened with an extraction solvent comprised of 50% acetonitrile and 50% methanol. A 10 cm × 10 cm disposable template was used to outline a 100 cm^2 sampling area. The sample area was wiped twice, once with the first Whatman filter, then again with the second Whatman filter. The two wipe samples were collectively analyzed by liquid chromatography mass spectrometry/mass spectrometry. All media and field blanks were below the LOD of 5 ng/sample for cyclophosphamide, 2 ng/sample for ifosfamide, and 7 ng/sample for doxorubicin. The sampling and analytical method was developed by Bureau Veritas North America. Results of a NIOSH stability study with cyclophosphamide and ifosfamide showed no degradation of recovery after 7 to 8 months for wipe samples stored frozen [Burr 2011a]. On the basis of these results, we do not suspect significant degradation of our field samples with respect to these two drugs. However, NIOSH chemists have observed in laboratory experiments that doxorubicin degraded after being frozen [Burr 2011b].

Biological Safety Cabinet Face Velocity

We used a TSI VelociCalc™ Model 8386 thermal anemometer (TSI, Shoreview, Minnesota) to measure the face velocity of the BSC where chemotherapy drugs were mixed and prepared. We took 65 measurements in a grid pattern (every 4 inches along the horizontal, every 2 inches along the vertical), and an arithmetic average was taken to determine the average face velocity.

References

Burr G [2011a]. E-mail on October 7, 2011, between G. Burr, Division of Surveillance, Hazard Evaluations and Field Studies and J. Pretty, Division of Applied Research and Technology, National Institute for Occupational Safety and Health, Centers for Disease Control and Prevention, U.S. Department of Health and Human Services.

Burr G [2011b]. Personal communication on September 29, 2011, between G. Burr, Division of Surveillance, Hazard Evaluations and Field Studies and J. Pretty, Division of Applied Research and Technology, National Institute for Occupational Safety and Health, Centers for Disease Control and Prevention, U.S. Department of Health and Human Services.

In evaluating the hazards posed by workplace exposures, NIOSH investigators use both mandatory (legally enforceable) and recommended OELs for chemical, physical, and biological agents as a guide for making recommendations. OELs have been developed by federal agencies and safety and health organizations to prevent the occurrence of adverse health effects from workplace exposures. Generally, OELs suggest levels of exposure that most employees may be exposed to for up to 10 hours per day, 40 hours per week, for a working lifetime, without experiencing adverse health effects. However, not all employees will be protected from adverse health effects even if their exposures are maintained below these levels. A small percentage may experience adverse health effects because of individual susceptibility, a pre-existing medical condition, and/or a hypersensitivity (allergy). In addition, some hazardous substances may act in combination with other workplace exposures, the general environment, or with medications or personal habits of the employee to produce adverse health effects even if the occupational exposures are controlled at the level set by the exposure limit. Also, some substances can be absorbed by direct contact with the skin and mucous membranes in addition to being inhaled, which contributes to the individual's overall exposure.

Most OELs are expressed as a TWA exposure. A TWA refers to the average exposure during a normal 8- to 10-hour workday. Some chemical substances and physical agents have recommended STEL or ceiling values where adverse health effects are caused by exposures over a short period. Unless otherwise noted, the STEL is a 15-minute TWA exposure that should not be exceeded at any time during a workday, and the ceiling limit is an exposure that should not be exceeded at any time.

In the United States, OELs have been established by federal agencies, professional organizations, state and local governments, and other entities. Some OELs are legally enforceable limits, while others are recommendations. The U.S. Department of Labor OSHA PELs (29 CFR 1910 [general industry]; 29 CFR 1926 [construction industry]; and 29 CFR 1917 [maritime industry]) are legal limits enforceable in workplaces covered under the Occupational Safety and Health Act of 1970. NIOSH RELs are recommendations based on a critical review of the scientific and technical information available on a given hazard and the adequacy of methods to identify and control the hazard. NIOSH RELs can be found in the *NIOSH Pocket Guide to Chemical Hazards* [NIOSH 2010]. NIOSH also recommends different types of risk management practices (e.g., engineering controls, safe work practices, employee education/training, personal protective equipment, and exposure and medical monitoring) to minimize the risk of exposure and adverse health effects from these hazards. Other OELs that are commonly used and cited in the United States include the TLVs recommended by ACGIH, a professional organization, and the WEELs recommended by the American Industrial Hygiene Association, another professional organization. The TLVs and WEELs are developed by committee members of these associations from a review of the published, peer-reviewed literature. They are not consensus standards. ACGIH TLVs are considered voluntary exposure guidelines for use by industrial hygienists and others trained in this discipline "to assist in the control of health hazards" [ACGIH 2011]. WEELs have been established for some chemicals "when no other legal or authoritative limits exist" [AIHA 2011].

Outside the United States, OELs have been established by various agencies and organizations and include both legal and recommended limits. The Institut für Arbeitsschutz der Deutschen Gesetzlichen Unfallversicherung (IFA, Institute for Occupational Safety and Health of the German Social Accident Insurance) maintains a database of international OELs from European Union member states, Canada (Québec), Japan, Switzerland, and the United States. The database, available at http://www.dguv.de/ifa/en/gestis/limit_values/index.jsp, contains international limits for over 1,500 hazardous substances and is updated periodically.

Employers should understand that not all hazardous chemicals have specific OSHA PELs, and for some agents the legally enforceable and recommended limits may not reflect current health-based information. However, an employer is still required by OSHA to protect its employees from hazards even in the absence of a specific OSHA PEL. OSHA requires an employer to furnish employees a place of employment free from recognized hazards that cause or are likely to cause death or serious physical harm [Occupational Safety and Health Act of 1970 (Public Law 91–596, sec. 5(a)(1))]. Thus, NIOSH investigators encourage employers to make use of other OELs when making risk assessments and risk management decisions to best protect the health of their employees. NIOSH investigators also encourage the use of the traditional hierarchy of controls approach to eliminate or minimize identified workplace hazards. This includes, in order of preference, the use of (1) substitution or elimination of the hazardous agent, (2) engineering controls (e.g., local exhaust ventilation, process enclosure, dilution ventilation), (3) administrative controls (e.g., limiting time of exposure, employee training, work practice changes, medical surveillance), and (4) personal protective equipment (e.g , respiratory protection, gloves, eye protection, hearing protection). Control banding, a qualitative risk assessment and risk management tool, is a complementary approach to protecting employee health that focuses resources on exposure controls by describing how a risk needs to be managed. Information on control banding is available at http://www.cdc.gov/niosh/topics/ctrlbanding/. This approach can be applied in situations where OELs have not been established or can be used to supplement the OELs, when available.

Below we provide the OELs and surface contamination limits for the compounds we measured, as well as a discussion of the potential health effects from exposure to these compounds.

Platinum-containing Chemotherapy Drugs

Platinum-containing chemotherapy drugs include cisplatin, oxiplatin, and carboplatin, among others. OSHA and NIOSH have not established OELs for platinum-containing chemotherapy drugs either as a group or as individual agents. However, these drugs can be considered individually based on their adverse health effects, carcinogenicity, teratogenicity, and other factors. For example, cisplatin is categorized at a Group 2A Carcinogen, meaning that there is inadequate evidence to designate it as a human carcinogen [IARC 2004].

Cyclophosphamide

Although OSHA and NIOSH have not established OELs for cyclophosphamide, it has been categorized as a Group 1 Carcinogen (carcinogenic to humans) by IARC [IARC 1998]. It metabolizes in the body to acrolein, which can cause adverse effects in the bladder.

Cyclophosphamide is a chemotherapy drug that is used for a wide range of neoplastic diseases such as breast and lung cancer, pediatric malignancies, leukemia, and lymphomas. It can be prescribed as a single drug or in combination with other chemotherapy drugs and can be administered via oral tablets or intravenously.

Cyclophosphamide is normally found in a white powder form for chemical stability and is typically brought into liquid solution by the addition of water and infused with sodium chloride, glucose, or glucose/saline solutions. Once in solution, it is recommended that cyclophosphamide be administered to the patient within 8 hours or stored cold (but not frozen) to prevent degradation. The surface wipe samples collected during this evaluation for cyclophosphamide, (as well as for ifosfamide and doxorubicin) were shipped cold from the field to the NIOSH laboratory. These wipe samples were then kept frozen for approximately 7 months pending development of an analytical method. There are currently no OELs for cyclophosphamide. However, because of its carcinogenic nature, exposures to cyclophosphamide should be controlled to the lowest achievable levels.

Ifosfamide

Ifosfamide is a chemotherapy drug that is used for a wide range of neoplastic diseases including ovary, testes, lung, breast, and soft-tissue sarcomas. It can be prescribed as a single drug or in combination with other chemotherapy drugs and can be administered via either oral tablets or intravenously. Ifosfamide is normally found in a white powder form for chemical stability and is normally brought into solution by the addition of water and infused with sodium chloride, glucose, or glucose/saline solutions.

Ifosfamide is a not designated as carcinogenic to humans by IARC, OSHA, or NIOSH. It has been reported to be mutagenic in bacterial cells through the Ames test. Ifosfamide metabolizes in the body to acrolein, which can cause adverse effects in the bladder. There are currently no OELs for ifosfamide.

Doxorubicin

Doxorubicin is a chemotherapy drug that is used for neoplastic diseases including leukemia, soft-tissue sarcomas, and solid tumors such as breast and lung cancer. It can be prescribed singly or in combination with other chemotherapy drugs and can be administered via oral tablets or intravenously. It is categorized as a Group 2A Carcinogen [IARC 1987], meaning that there is inadequate evidence to designate it as a human carcinogen.

Chemotherapy Drugs in Health Care Settings

Occupational exposures to chemotherapy drugs may occur through inhalation, skin contact, skin absorption, ingestion, or injection. Inhalation and skin contact/absorption are the most likely routes of exposure, but unintentional ingestion from hand to mouth contact and unintentional injection through a needlestick or sharps injury are also possible [Duvall and Baumann 1980; Black and Presson 1997; Schreiber et al. 2003].

Protection from chemotherapy drug exposures depends on safety programs established by employers and followed by employees. Factors that affect employee exposures include drug handling circumstances (preparation, administration, or disposal), amount of drug prepared, frequency and duration of drug handling, potential for absorption, use of ventilated cabinets, PPE, and work practices. The chance that an employee will experience adverse effects from chemotherapy drugs increases with the amount and frequency of exposure and the lack of proper work practices [NIOSH 2004].

Studies have associated workplace exposures to chemotherapy drugs with acute health effects, primarily in nurses. These included hair loss, headaches, acute irritation, and/or hypersensitivity [Valanis et al. 1993a; Valanis et al. 1993b]. The major reproductive effects found in these studies were increased fetal loss [Selevan et al. 1985; Stücker et al. 1990], congenital malformations depending on the length of exposure [Hemminki et al. 1985], low birth weight and congenital abnormalities [Peelen et al. 1999], and infertility [Valanis et al. 1999].

Several reports have addressed the relationship of cancer occurrence to health care employees' exposures to chemotherapy drugs [NIOSH 2004]. A significantly increased risk of leukemia has been reported among oncology nurses identified in the Danish cancer registry for the period 1943–1987 [Skov et al. 1992]. The same group [Skov et al. 1990] found an increased, but not significant, risk of leukemia in physicians employed for at least 6 months in a department where patients were treated with chemotherapy drugs.

References

ACGIH [2011]. 2011 TLVs® and BEIs®: threshold limit values for chemical substances and physical agents and biological exposure indices. Cincinnati, OH: American Conference of Governmental Industrial Hygienists.

AIHA [2011]. AIHA 2011 Emergency response planning guidelines (ERPG) & workplace environmental exposure levels (WEEL) handbook. Fairfax, VA: American Industrial Hygiene Association.

Black LA, Presson AC [1997]. Hazardous drugs. Occup Med: State of the Art Rev 12(4):669–685.

CFR. Code of Federal Regulations. Washington, DC: U.S. Government Printing Office, Office of the Federal Register.

Duvall E, Baumann B [1980]. An unusual accident during the administration of chemotherapy. Cancer Nurs 3(4):305–306.

Harrison BR [2001]. Risks of handling cytotoxic drugs. In: Perry MC, ed. The chemotherapy source book. 3rd ed. Philadelphia, PA: Lippincott, Williams and Wilkins, pp. 566–582.

Hemminki K, Kyyrönen P, Lindbohm M-L [1985]. Spontaneous abortions and malformations in the offspring of nurses exposed to anesthetic gases, cytostatic drugs, and other potential hazards in hospitals, based on registered information of outcome. J Epidemiol Commun Health 39:141–147.

IARC [1987]. Overall Evaluations of Carcinogenicity: an updating of IARC Monographs Volumes 1 to 42. Lyon: IARC monographs on the evaluation of carcinogenic risks to humans; Supplement 7. International Agency for Research on Cancer.

IARC [1998]. Some antineoplastic and immunosuppressive agents. Lyon: IARC monographs on the evaluation of carcinogenic risks to humans, vol 26. International Agency for Research on Cancer.

IARC [2004]. IARC monographs on the evaluation of the carcinogenic risk of chemicals to humans. Lyons, France: World Health Organization, International Agency for Research on Cancer. [http://monographs iarc.fr/]. Date accessed: March 2012.

NIOSH [2004]. NIOSH alert: preventing occupational exposure to antineoplastic and other hazardous drugs in health care settings. Cincinnati, OH: U.S. Department of Health and Human Services, Centers for Disease Control and Prevention, National Institute for Occupational Safety and Health, DHHS (NIOSH) Publication No. 2004-165.

NIOSH [2010]. NIOSH pocket guide to chemical hazards. Cincinnati, OH: U.S. Department of Health and Human Services, Centers for Disease Control and Prevention, National Institute for Occupational Safety and Health, DHHS (NIOSH) Publication No. 2010-168c. [http://www.cdc.gov/niosh/npg/]. Date accessed: March 2012.

Peelen S, Roeleveld N, Heederik D, Krombout H, de Kort W [1999]. Toxic effects on reproduction in hospital personnel (in Dutch). Netherlands: Elsevier.

Schreiber C, Radon K, Pethran A, Schierl R, Hauff K, Grimm C-H, Boos K-S, Nowak D. [2003]. Uptake of antineoplastic agents in pharmacy personnel. Part 2: study of work-related risk factors. Int Arch Occup Environ Health 76(1):11–16.

Selevan SG, Lindbohm M-L, Hornung RW, Hemminki K [1985]. A study of occupa¬tional exposure to antineoplastic drugs and fetal loss in nurses. N Engl J Med 313(19):1173–1178.

Skov T, Lynge E, Maarup B, Olsen J, Rørth M, Winthereik H [1990]. Risk for physicians handling antineoplastic drugs [letter to the editor]. Lancet 336(8728):1446.

Skov T, Maarup B, Olsen J, Rørth M, Winthereik H, Lynge E [1992]. Leukaemia and reproductive outcome among nurses handling antineoplastic drugs. Br J Ind Med 49(12):855–861.

Stücker I, Caillard J-F, Collin R, Gout M, Poyen D, Hémon D [1990]. Risk of spontaneous abortion among nurses handling antineoplastic drugs. Scand J Work Environ Health 16(2):102–107.

Valanis BG, Vollmer WM, Labuhn KT, Glass AG [1993a]. Acute symptoms associated with antineoplastic drug handling among nurses. Cancer Nurs 16(4):288–295.

Valanis BG, Vollmer WM, Labuhn KT, Glass AG [1993b]. Association of antineoplastic drug handling with acute adverse effects in pharmacy personnel. Am J Hosp Pharm 50(3):455–462.

Valanis B, Vollmer WM, Steele P [1999]. Occupational exposure to antineoplastic agents: self-reported miscarriages and stillbirths among nurses and pharmacists. J Occup Environ Med 41(8):632–638.

APPENDIX C: TABLES

Table C1. Platinum-containing chemotherapy drugs in surface wipe samples collected in September 2009 and November 2010

Location	Description	Results ng/100 cm^2	
		September 2009†	November 2010‡
Clinic pharmacy	Countertop in front of prepared drugs	48	3.4
	On top of chemo-waste container (gowns/jackets)	(3.4)	NS
	Middle of chemotherapy preparation hood	14	12
	On floor in front of prepared drugs	91	3.3
	Inside empty pharmacy cooler	(2.0)	(0.48)
	Outside of oxaliplatin bag	ND	NS
	On floor in front of pharmacy hood	(8.5)	5.7
	Inside the door handle exiting pharmacy*	(1.6)	NS
	Countertop underneath oxaliplatin bag	(7.2)	NS
	Next to sink	11	5.0
Left treatment room	Arm of first chair	(2.1)	2.9
	Under IV stand next to first chair	(1.3)	2.1
	Keypad of IV pump next to first chair	(1.5)	(0.77)
	Table to left of first chair	(0.85)	NS
	Supply area sink (left side) behind nurse station	(2.3)	NS
	"Quiet Room" area on the arm of chair	(1.5)	NS
	Handle of faucet*	ND	NS
Nurse station	Desk on the right side of keyboard	ND	(0.38)
Exam room #4	Countertop to the right of sink	ND	ND
Dictation room	Desk on the right side of keyboard	ND	ND
Waiting room	Table next to first chair	ND	ND
Checkout	First desk on right	ND	ND
Right treatment room	Under IV stand on floor	(1.4)	5.9
	Arm of first chair	(1.0)	0.97
	Food rollaway table	ND	(0.77)
	Countertop next to sink in bedroom	(1.6)	13
Injection room	Side table next to recliner	NS	(0.57)
Room behind nurse station	On edge of countertop near wastebasket	NS	1.4

*Estimated 100 cm^2 sampling area
†September 2009: LOD = 0.7 ng platinum/sample and LOQ = 9.8 ng platinum/sample
‡November 2010: LOD = 0.3 ng platinum/sample and LOQ = 0.84 ng platinum/sample
( ) Sample results in parentheses were between the LOD and the LOQ, meaning that they have more uncertainty associated with them.
ND = not detected (below the LOD)
NS = location was not sampled

Table C2. Cyclophosphamide in surface wipe samples collected in November 2010

Room	Location	Results reported in ng/100 cm^2					
		Day 1	Day 2		Day 3		Day 4
		PM	AM	PM	AM	PM	AM
Clinic pharmacy	Prepared drugs countertop	ND	ND	ND	ND	ND	ND
	BSC work surface	ND	NS	NS	NS	NS	NS
	Floor in front of prepared drugs	36	(13)	20	(13)	(16)	18
	Inside empty cooler	ND	NS	NS	NS	NS	NS
	On floor in front of BSC	41	59	56	63	69	50
	Countertop next to sink	ND	ND	ND	ND	ND	ND
Left treatment room	Arm of first chair	ND	ND	ND	ND	(7.8)	ND
	Under IV stand next to first chair	33	43	28,000	470	120	54
	Keypad of IV pump next to chair*	ND	ND	ND	ND	ND	ND
Nurse station	Desk near keyboard	ND	ND	ND	ND	ND	ND
Exam room 4	Countertop next to sink	ND	ND	ND	ND	ND	ND
Dictation room	Desk near computer keyboard	ND	ND	ND	ND	ND	ND
Waiting room	Coffee table	ND	NS	NS	NS	NS	NS
Checkout	Desk surface on right	(15)	22	(5.7)	(12)	(17)	(8.0)
Right treatment room	Under IV stand	21	NS	NS	NS	NS	NS
	Arm of first chair	ND	NS	NS	NS	NS	NS
	Food rollaway table	ND	NS	NS	NS	NS	NS
	Countertop next to sink	ND	ND	ND	ND	ND	ND
Room behind nurse station	Desk on countertop	ND	ND	ND	ND	ND	ND
Injection room	Side table next to recliner	ND	ND	ND	ND	ND	ND

*Estimated 100 cm^2 sampling area
AM = Sample collected in the morning prior to any chemotherapy drug administration
PM = Sample collected at the end of the day prior to housecleaning activities
LOD = 5 ng/sample
LOQ = 17 ng/sample
ND = not detected (below the LOD)
NS = location was not sampled
( ) Sample results in parentheses were between the LOD and the LOQ, meaning that they have more uncertainty associated with them.

Table C3. Ifosfamide in surface wipe samples collected in November 2010

Room	Location	Results reported in ng/100 cm²					
		Day 1	Day 2		Day 3		Day 4
		PM	AM	PM	AM	PM	AM
Clinic pharmacy	Prepared drugs countertop	ND	ND	ND	ND	ND	ND
	BSC work surface	ND	NS	NS	NS	NS	NS
	Floor in front of prepared drugs	ND	ND	ND	ND	ND	ND
	Inside empty cooler	ND	NS	NS	NS	NS	NS
	On floor in front of BSC	ND	ND	ND	(2.0)	(2.7)	ND
	Countertop next to sink	ND	ND	ND	ND	ND	ND
Left treatment room	Arm of first chair	ND	ND	ND	ND	ND	ND
	Under IV stand next to first chair	ND	ND	ND	ND	ND	ND
	Keypad of IV pump next to chair*	ND	ND	ND	ND	ND	ND
Nurse station	Desk near keyboard	ND	ND	ND	ND	ND	ND
Exam room 4	Countertop next to sink	ND	ND	ND	ND	ND	ND
Dictation room	Desk near computer keyboard	ND	ND	ND	ND	ND	ND
Waiting room	Coffee table	ND	NS	NS	NS	NS	NS
Checkout	Desk surface on right	ND	ND	ND	ND	ND	ND
Right treatment room	Under IV stand	ND	NS	NS	NS	NS	NS
	Arm of first chair	ND	NS	NS	NS	NS	NS
	Food rollaway table	ND	NS	NS	NS	NS	NS
	Countertop next to sink	ND	ND	ND	ND	ND	ND
Room behind nurse station	Desk on countertop	ND	ND	ND	ND	ND	ND
Injection room	Side table next to recliner	ND	ND	ND	ND	ND	ND

*Estimated 100 cm² sampling area
AM = Sample collected in the morning prior to any chemotherapy drug administration
PM = Sample collected at the end of the day prior to housecleaning activities
LOD = 2 ng/sample
LOQ = 7.3 ng/sample
ND = not detected (below the LOD)
NS = location was not sampled
( ) Sample results in parentheses were between the LOD and the LOQ, meaning that they have more uncertainty associated with them.

Acknowledgments and Availability of Report

The Hazard Evaluations and Technical Assistance Branch (HETAB) of the National Institute for Occupational Safety and Health (NIOSH) conducts field investigations of possible health hazards in the workplace. These investigations are conducted under the authority of Section 20(a)(6) of the Occupational Safety and Health Act of 1970, 29 U.S.C. 669(a)(6) which authorizes the Secretary of Health and Human Services, following a written request from any employer or authorized representative of employees, to determine whether any substance normally found in the place of employment has potentially toxic effects in such concentrations as used or found. HETAB also provides, upon request, technical and consultative assistance to federal, state, and local agencies; labor; industry; and other groups or individuals to control occupational health hazards and to prevent related trauma and disease.

Mention of any company or product does not constitute endorsement by NIOSH. In addition, citations to websites external to NIOSH do not constitute NIOSH endorsement of the sponsoring organizations or their programs or products. Furthermore, NIOSH is not responsible for the content of these websites. All Web addresses referenced in this document were accessible as of the publication date.

This report was prepared by James Couch and Christine West of HETAB, Division of Surveillance, Hazard Evaluations and Field Studies. Industrial hygiene field assistance was provided by Scott Brueck and Bradley King. Industrial hygiene equipment and logistical support was provided by Donald Booher and Karl Feldmann. Health communication assistance was provided by Stefanie Evans. Editorial assistance was provided by Ellen Galloway. Desktop publishing was performed by Greg Hartle and Mary Winfree.

Copies of this report have been sent to employee and management representatives at the clinic, the state health department, and the Occupational Safety and Health Administration Regional Office. This report is not copyrighted and may be freely reproduced. The report may be viewed and printed at http://www.cdc.gov/niosh/hhe/. Copies may be purchased from the National Technical Information Service at 5825 Port Royal Road, Springfield, Virginia 22161.

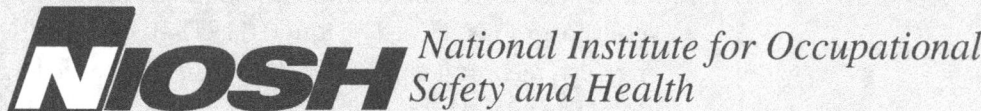

National Institute for Occupational Safety and Health

Delivering on the Nation's promise: Safety and health at work for all people through research and prevention.

To receive NIOSH documents or information about occupational safety and health topics, contact NIOSH at:

1-800-CDC-INFO (1-800-232-4636)

TTY: 1-888-232-6348

E-mail: cdcinfo@cdc.gov

or visit the NIOSH web site at: **www.cdc.gov/niosh.**

For a monthly update on news at NIOSH, subscribe to NIOSH eNews by visiting **www.cdc.gov/niosh/eNews.**

SAFER • HEALTHIER • PEOPLE™

www.ingramcontent.com/pod-product-compliance
Lightning Source LLC
Chambersburg PA
CBHW080933290526

45795CB00007BA/2732